LIVING WITH COPD

Strategies To Breathe Easier Everyday

Jason Moore

Disclaimer

The information presented in this book is intended for educational and informational purposes only and should not be considered as medical advice. While every effort has been made to ensure the accuracy of the content, the authors and publishers are not healthcare professionals and cannot guarantee that the information provided will be suitable for every individual. Readers are strongly encouraged to consult with their healthcare provider or a qualified medical professional before making any changes to their treatment plan, medication, or lifestyle. COPD is a complex medical condition, and individualized care is essential for managing symptoms and maintaining quality of life. This book does not replace professional medical advice, diagnosis, or treatment. If you experience a medical emergency or significant changes in your condition, seek immediate medical attention. The authors and publishers disclaim any liability for any adverse outcomes resulting from the use or application of the information contained in this book.

CONTENTS

INTRODUCTION

Living with Chronic Obstructive Pulmonary Disease (COPD) can be challenging, but it doesn't mean you have to sacrifice a fulfilling and meaningful life. Whether you were recently diagnosed or have been navigating this condition for years, this e-book is designed to provide you with practical strategies, insightful advice, and compassionate encouragement.

COPD is a progressive lung disease that affects millions of people worldwide, presenting unique physical, emotional, and social challenges. While the road ahead may feel uncertain, knowledge and preparation are powerful tools. This e-book offers a roadmap to help you better understand COPD, manage your symptoms, and improve your overall quality of life.

You'll discover:

- What COPD is and how it affects your body.
- Ways to communicate effectively with your healthcare team.
- Tips for improving your breathing and conserving energy.
- Strategies for maintaining mental well-being and staying active.
- Tools for building a support system to keep you motivated.

Living with COPD doesn't mean giving up—it means adapting, thriving, and taking control where you can. Through a blend of medical insights, lifestyle tips, and personal stories, this e-book empowers you to face the challenges of COPD with resilience and hope.

Let's take this journey together, one step at a time, and discover how you can embrace life fully while managing COPD.

CHAPTER 1: UNDERSTANDING COPD

The Science of COPD

Chronic Obstructive Pulmonary Disease (COPD) is a progressive lung condition that makes it difficult to breathe. It encompasses two primary conditions: chronic bronchitis, characterized by long-term inflammation of the airways, and emphysema, which involves damage to the tiny air sacs (alveoli) in the lungs.

In healthy lungs, airways are clear, and oxygen easily passes into the bloodstream through the alveoli. With COPD, inflammation, mucus buildup, and structural damage obstruct airflow, reducing the lungs' efficiency. This leads to symptoms such as shortness of breath, chronic cough, and a feeling of tightness in the chest.

COPD is progressive, meaning it worsens over time, but with proper management, many people live fulfilling lives. Understanding how COPD affects the body is the first step in taking control.

Causes and Risk Factors

- Smoking

Smoking is the leading cause of COPD, accounting for approximately 75% of cases. The toxins in cigarette smoke irritate the lungs, causing long-term damage. While not all smokers develop COPD, those with prolonged exposure to tobacco are at higher risk.

- Environmental Factors

Prolonged exposure to pollutants such as industrial fumes, dust, and chemical vapors can contribute to COPD. Indoor air pollution, like smoke from burning fuel for cooking or heating, also poses a risk, particularly in low-income areas worldwide.

- Genetics

A hereditary condition called alpha-1 antitrypsin deficiency increases susceptibility to COPD, even in nonsmokers. This rare genetic factor can lead to early-onset emphysema.

- Age and Gender

COPD is more common in people over 40, as lung function naturally declines with age. Historically, men were more likely to develop COPD, but rates among women have increased due to rising smoking rates and increased exposure to environmental risks.

Stages of COPD

COPD progresses in four stages, as measured by spirometry (a test to assess lung function):

- Mild (Stage 1)

- Symptoms: Chronic cough and minor breathlessness.
- Lung Function: Slight reduction, but most people function normally.
- Moderate (Stage 2)

- Symptoms: Increased breathlessness, wheezing, and frequent infections.
- Lung Function: Noticeable decline; medical attention often begins here.
- Severe (Stage 3)

- Symptoms: Difficulty with daily activities, fatigue, and more severe flare-ups.
- Lung Function: Significant reduction; oxygen therapy may be required.
- Very Severe (Stage 4)

- Symptoms: Extreme shortness of breath, even at rest.
- Lung Function: Minimal; daily life is heavily impacted.

How COPD is Diagnosed

- Medical History

Your healthcare provider will ask about smoking habits, exposure to pollutants, family history, and symptoms. Chronic cough, excessive mucus production, and shortness of breath are red flags.

•	Spirometry
This simple breathing test measures how much air you can exhale forcefully and how quickly. It's the gold standard for diagnosing and staging COPD.

•	Imaging Tests

•	Chest X-ray: Detects signs of emphysema or other lung issues.
•	CT Scan: Provides a more detailed view to identify damage or infections.
•	Blood Tests
A blood test for alpha-1 antitrypsin deficiency may be recommended, especially if there's no smoking history or if COPD develops at a young age.

Understanding Your Diagnosis
Receiving a COPD diagnosis can be overwhelming, but it's important to see it as an opportunity to take charge of your health. Early diagnosis allows for better management of symptoms and slows disease progression.
•	Accepting the Reality: Acknowledge the diagnosis without blame. Many factors, including genetics and environment, contribute to COPD.
•	Learning About the Disease: The more you know, the better equipped you are to manage it.
•	Partnering with Your Healthcare Team: Work with your doctors and specialists to create a personalized treatment plan.
Remember, COPD doesn't define you. With proper care, support, and lifestyle adjustments, you can lead a fulfilling and active life.

CHAPTER 2: BUILDING YOUR COPD CARE TEAM

Living with COPD requires a comprehensive and collaborative approach to care. Building a strong healthcare team and maintaining clear communication with them can significantly improve your quality of life. This chapter will guide you in assembling and working with your care team to ensure your needs are met effectively.

Who's on Your Care Team?

Your COPD care team is made up of various professionals, each contributing expertise to help manage different aspects of the disease. Here's who you might have on your team:

- Primary Care Physician (PCP)

- Often the first point of contact for managing your overall health.
- Monitors your general well-being and coordinates with specialists.
- Pulmonologist

- A lung specialist who diagnoses, treats, and monitors your COPD.
- Provides guidance on medications, oxygen therapy, and other treatments.
- Respiratory Therapist

- Teaches you breathing techniques and exercises to improve lung function.
- Offers support for using inhalers, nebulizers, and supplemental oxygen.
- Pharmacist

- Ensures you understand your medications, including

proper usage and potential side effects.
•	Helps manage drug interactions and offers advice on over-the-counter options.
•	Dietitian or Nutritionist

•	Advises on dietary choices to support lung health and maintain a healthy weight.
•	Addresses nutritional challenges related to COPD, such as loss of appetite or fatigue.
•	Physical Therapist

•	Develops exercise programs tailored to your abilities.
•	Focuses on improving strength, endurance, and overall fitness.
•	Mental Health Professional

•	Provides counseling or therapy to help cope with the emotional challenges of COPD.
•	Offers strategies for managing anxiety, depression, or stress.
•	Social Worker or Case Manager

•	Assists with navigating insurance, disability benefits, and access to community resources.
•	Provides support for financial or logistical concerns.

Communication is Key
Clear and open communication with your care team is essential for effective management of COPD. Here's how to ensure your needs and concerns are understood:
•	Be Honest About Symptoms

•	Share all symptoms, even minor ones, as they may indicate changes in your condition.
•	Keep a symptom journal to track patterns or triggers.
•	Ask Questions

•	Don't hesitate to ask for clarification about your treatment plan or medications.

- Prepare a list of questions before appointments to ensure you cover everything.
- Provide Updates

- Inform your team about any changes in symptoms, lifestyle, or challenges you face.
- Share feedback on how treatments are working or any side effects you experience.
- Advocate for Yourself

- If something isn't working or you feel uncertain, speak up.
- Request second opinions or additional resources if needed.

Establishing a Partnership with Your Care Team
Managing COPD is a team effort. Here are some tips for building a strong partnership with your healthcare providers:
- Set Clear Goals

- Work with your care team to establish realistic short-term and long-term goals, such as improving stamina, reducing flare-ups, or quitting smoking.
- Follow Through on Recommendations

- Adhere to prescribed medications, therapies, and lifestyle changes.
- Commit to attending follow-up appointments and routine check-ups.
- Stay Informed

- Learn about COPD through reliable sources and bring new questions or insights to your team.
- Be cautious about misinformation and discuss any concerns with your healthcare providers.
- Involve Loved Ones

- Bring a trusted family member or friend to appointments for additional support and to help remember details.
- Involving loved ones helps them understand your condition and how they can assist.

Maximizing Care Between Appointments

Your healthcare team isn't just for emergencies or scheduled visits. Here's how to make the most of their expertise between appointments:

•	Leverage Technology

•	Use patient portals to communicate with your doctors, request refills, or review test results.
•	Consider apps designed to track medications, symptoms, and activity levels.
•	Emergency Preparedness

•	Know who to contact in case of a flare-up or emergency.
•	Keep a written action plan, including medication lists and key phone numbers.
•	Stay Connected

•	Don't wait for appointments if you have pressing questions or concerns.
•	Many providers offer telemedicine options for quicker consultations.

Building Trust and Confidence

Trust is the foundation of a successful care partnership. By actively participating in your care and maintaining honest communication, you'll foster a strong relationship with your team.

•	Trust Their Expertise: Remember that your team is dedicated to your well-being.
•	Take Responsibility: Stay proactive in managing your condition through self-care and adherence to their advice.
•	Celebrate Successes: Share progress with your care team to reinforce the positive impact of their efforts and your own.

A well-rounded care team and open communication can make a significant difference in managing COPD. You're not alone on this journey—your team is there to support you every step of the way.

CHAPTER 3: MEDICAL MANAGEMENT OF COPD

Medical management is a cornerstone of living well with Chronic Obstructive Pulmonary Disease (COPD). The right combination of medications, therapies, and regular monitoring can alleviate symptoms, reduce flare-ups, and improve overall quality of life. This chapter outlines the tools and treatments your healthcare team may use to help you manage COPD effectively.

Medications for COPD

Medications are essential for managing symptoms, preventing complications, and slowing the progression of COPD. Depending on the severity of your condition, your doctor may prescribe one or more of the following:

- Bronchodilators

- Purpose: Relax the muscles around your airways, making it easier to breathe.
- Types: Short-acting (used for quick relief) and long-acting (used for maintenance).
- Examples: Albuterol (short-acting), Salmeterol (long-acting).
- Inhaled Corticosteroids

- Purpose: Reduce inflammation in the airways to prevent exacerbations.
- Examples: Fluticasone, Budesonide.
- Considerations: Typically used for moderate to severe COPD or in combination with   bronchodilators.
- Combination Inhalers

- Purpose: Combine bronchodilators and corticosteroids in a single device for convenience and enhanced effectiveness.
- Examples: Advair, Symbicort.

- Phosphodiesterase-4 (PDE4) Inhibitors

- Purpose: Reduce inflammation and relax the airways.
- Example: Roflumilast.
- Usage: For severe COPD with chronic bronchitis.
- Mucolytics

- Purpose: Thin mucus, making it easier to clear from your airways.
- Examples: Carbocysteine, N-acetylcysteine.
- Antibiotics and Antivirals

- Purpose: Treat or prevent infections that can worsen COPD symptoms.
- Usage: Often prescribed during exacerbations or to manage frequent respiratory infections.

Oxygen Therapy
For those with advanced COPD, oxygen therapy can be life-changing. When your lungs can't provide enough oxygen to your blood, supplemental oxygen ensures your body gets the support it needs.
- When is it Prescribed?

- Oxygen therapy is recommended if blood oxygen levels are consistently low, as measured by pulse oximetry or arterial blood gas tests.
- Types of Delivery Systems

- Nasal cannula (most common).
- Face masks for higher oxygen needs.
- Portable oxygen concentrators for mobility.
- Safety Tips

- Avoid smoking or open flames near oxygen equipment.
- Regularly maintain equipment to ensure it functions properly.

Pulmonary Rehabilitation

Pulmonary rehabilitation is a structured program combining exercise, education, and support designed to improve your physical and emotional well-being.
- What's Included?

- Supervised exercise to improve strength and stamina.
- Breathing techniques, such as pursed-lip breathing.
- Education on managing symptoms, medications, and nutrition.
- Benefits

- Enhances your ability to perform daily activities.
- Reduces symptoms like breathlessness and fatigue.
- Improves mental health and confidence.

Vaccinations and Preventive Care

COPD increases your vulnerability to respiratory infections, which can lead to dangerous exacerbations. Staying up to date on vaccinations is critical:
- Flu Vaccine

- Annual flu shots protect against seasonal influenza, a common trigger for COPD flare-ups.
- Pneumococcal Vaccine

- Protects against pneumonia, which can cause severe complications for people with COPD.
- COVID-19 Vaccine and Boosters

- Reduces the risk of severe illness from COVID-19, which can exacerbate COPD symptoms.
- Tdap Vaccine

- Protects against pertussis (whooping cough), tetanus, and diphtheria.

Monitoring Your Progress

Regular check-ups and monitoring are essential to track the progression of COPD and adjust treatments as needed.

- Routine Tests

- Spirometry: Measures lung function over time.
- Pulse Oximetry: Monitors oxygen levels in your blood.
- Arterial Blood Gas Test: Provides a detailed analysis of oxygen and carbon dioxide levels.
- Action Plans

- Work with your doctor to develop a written action plan for managing symptoms and flare-ups.
- Include instructions for medications, when to seek medical help, and steps for emergencies.
- Self-Monitoring

- Keep track of symptoms, medication usage, and triggers in a journal or app.
- Early recognition of changes can prevent exacerbations.

Surgical Options for Severe COPD

In advanced cases where medications and therapies are insufficient, surgical interventions may be considered.

- Lung Volume Reduction Surgery (LVRS)

- Removes damaged lung tissue to allow healthier lung areas to function better.
- Bullectomy

- Removes large air pockets (bullae) that can interfere with breathing.
- Lung Transplant

- A last-resort option for individuals with end-stage COPD who meet strict criteria.

The Importance of Adherence

Consistently following your treatment plan is crucial for managing COPD effectively. Skipping medications, neglecting therapy, or failing to attend appointments can lead to worsening symptoms and reduced quality of life.

- Tips for Staying on Track
- Set medication reminders on your phone.
- Use a pill organizer to avoid missed doses.
- Involve loved ones in your care for support and accountability.

Empowering Yourself Through Knowledge

Medical management is an evolving process that requires collaboration with your healthcare team. By understanding your treatment options, staying proactive, and following your plan, you can take control of your COPD and live life to its fullest.

CHAPTER 4: LIFESTYLE CHANGES FOR BETTER LIVING

Living with COPD involves more than just medical treatments. Your lifestyle plays a crucial role in managing symptoms, slowing disease progression, and improving your overall quality of life. By making intentional changes and adopting healthier habits, you can better cope with COPD and enjoy greater well-being.

Quitting Smoking: The Most Important Step
Smoking is the leading cause of COPD and continues to worsen symptoms and lung function over time. Quitting is the single most effective way to slow the progression of the disease.

- Why It's Critical to Quit

- Smoking damages the lungs, reduces oxygen levels, and exacerbates symptoms.
- Even reducing the number of cigarettes smoked per day can have significant benefits.
- Resources to Help You Quit

- Nicotine Replacement Therapy (NRT): Patches, gum, lozenges, or inhalers to reduce cravings.
- Medications: Prescription options like bupropion (Zyban) or varenicline (Chantix).
- Support Programs: Smoking cessation classes, hotlines, and online forums.
- Tips for Success

- Identify triggers and develop strategies to avoid them.
- Replace smoking with healthier habits, such as chewing gum or taking a walk.
- Celebrate milestones, like a week or month without smoking.

Managing Environmental Triggers

The environment around you can significantly impact your symptoms. Minimizing exposure to irritants helps reduce flare-ups and improves lung health.

*   Common Triggers

*   Air pollution, dust, and chemical fumes.
*   Secondhand smoke or strong odors from cleaning products and perfumes.
*   Pollen, pet dander, and other allergens.
*   Steps to Reduce Exposure

*   Use air purifiers and keep windows closed on high-pollution days.
*   Maintain a clean home by vacuuming and dusting regularly.
*   Avoid outdoor activities during high pollen seasons or extreme weather.
*   Workplace Adjustments

*   Discuss accommodations with your employer if your job involves exposure to harmful substances.

Nutrition and COPD

What you eat can directly affect your energy levels, lung function, and ability to fight infections. A balanced diet tailored to your needs is essential for managing COPD.

*   Nutritional Priorities

*   High-Protein Foods: Help maintain muscle strength (lean meats, fish, eggs, beans).
*   Fruits and Vegetables: Rich in antioxidants to support lung health.
*   Healthy Fats: Provide energy without overloading your digestive system (avocado, nuts, olive oil).
*   Foods to Avoid

*   Limit salt to prevent water retention and bloating.

- Avoid carbonated beverages, which can increase bloating and discomfort.
- Steer clear of processed and fried foods that may trigger inflammation.
- Meal Planning Tips

- Eat smaller, more frequent meals to avoid feeling too full, which can pressure the diaphragm.
- Stay hydrated by drinking water throughout the day to thin mucus.

Building an Active Lifestyle

Regular physical activity is essential for maintaining lung function, improving stamina, and boosting overall health. With COPD, the key is finding the right balance between activity and rest.

- Benefits of Exercise

- Strengthens respiratory muscles and improves oxygen efficiency.
- Reduces symptoms like shortness of breath and fatigue.
- Enhances mood and reduces anxiety or depression.
- Types of Activities to Consider

- Walking: A simple and effective way to stay active.
- Stretching: Improves flexibility and reduces muscle tension.
- Strength Training: Builds muscle to support daily activities.
- Breathing Exercises: Techniques like pursed-lip breathing or diaphragmatic breathing to improve oxygen flow.
- Tips for Exercising Safely

- Start slow and increase intensity gradually.
- Avoid overexertion—rest when needed.
- Exercise indoors during extreme weather conditions.

Getting Quality Sleep

COPD symptoms like shortness of breath, coughing, or discomfort can make restful sleep challenging. However, good sleep is vital for energy and overall health.

•	Improving Sleep Hygiene

•	Maintain a regular sleep schedule.
•	Create a comfortable sleeping environment with clean air and minimal noise.
•	Avoid caffeine or heavy meals close to bedtime.
•	Managing Nighttime Symptoms

•	Use extra pillows to elevate your head, which can ease breathing.
•	Follow your doctor's recommendations for nighttime oxygen therapy if prescribed.

Reducing Stress and Managing Mental Health
Living with COPD can be emotionally challenging, leading to anxiety, depression, or frustration. Prioritizing mental health is as important as managing physical symptoms.

•	Stress-Reduction Techniques

•	Practice mindfulness or meditation to stay calm and focused.
•	Engage in hobbies or activities that bring joy and relaxation.
•	Spend time in nature or with loved ones to uplift your mood.
•	Seeking Support

•	Talk to a counselor or therapist if you feel overwhelmed.
•	Join COPD support groups to connect with others facing similar challenges.
•	Mind-Body Practices

•	Try yoga or tai chi, which combine gentle movement with focused breathing.

The Power of Routine and Consistency

Establishing a routine can help you incorporate these lifestyle changes seamlessly into your daily life. Consistency is key for building habits that support long-term health.

- Create a Daily Schedule

- Include time for meals, medication, exercise, and rest.
- Set reminders for inhalers, supplements, or breathing exercises.
- Track Your Progress

- Use a journal or app to log symptoms, triggers, and improvements.
- Celebrate milestones, no matter how small, to stay motivated.

Conclusion

Lifestyle changes are not just about managing COPD—they are about reclaiming control over your health and enhancing your quality of life. By adopting healthier habits and making small, consistent changes, you can take meaningful steps toward feeling better every day.

Remember, change doesn't happen overnight. Be patient with yourself, and focus on progress rather than perfection.

CHAPTER 5: EXERCISE AND PHYSICAL ACTIVITY FOR COPD

Exercise is one of the most beneficial lifestyle changes you can make when living with COPD. While it might seem challenging at first, regular physical activity can improve lung function, reduce breathlessness, and enhance your overall well-being. This chapter will guide you on how to incorporate exercise into your life safely and effectively, regardless of your COPD stage.

The Importance of Exercise in COPD

Exercise is often overlooked by people with COPD, yet it plays a crucial role in managing the disease. Regular physical activity helps to:

- Improve Lung Efficiency

- Exercise strengthens the respiratory muscles, making it easier to breathe and improving oxygen exchange.
- Increases your ability to tolerate physical exertion without becoming overly breathless.
- Increase Muscle Strength and Endurance

- COPD can lead to muscle weakness due to inactivity, but regular exercise helps prevent muscle loss and improves strength.
- Enhanced endurance allows you to carry out daily activities with less fatigue.
- Boost Cardiovascular Health

- Exercise improves heart health, ensuring better blood circulation, which is essential for lung function and overall vitality.
- Reduce Symptoms

- Regular exercise helps reduce the feeling of breathlessness and can decrease the frequency and severity of flare-ups.

- It can also enhance your mood, combatting depression and anxiety often associated with chronic illness.

Types of Exercise for COPD

Not all exercises are created equal, and some are better suited for individuals with COPD than others. Here are a few types of exercise that can be beneficial:

- Aerobic Exercise (Cardio)

- Examples: Walking, cycling, swimming, or low-impact dance.
- Why It's Effective: Aerobic activities get your heart rate up, improving stamina and cardiovascular health. They also help increase lung capacity and oxygen delivery.
- How to Start: Begin with shorter sessions (5-10 minutes) and gradually increase duration as you build stamina.
- Strength Training (Resistance Exercise)

- Examples: Weight lifting, using resistance bands, or bodyweight exercises (e.g., squats, lunges, wall push-ups).
- Why It's Effective: Strength training increases muscle mass, which helps support better mobility and decreases fatigue. It also helps maintain balance and prevent falls.
- How to Start: Focus on small, controlled movements. Start with light weights or resistance bands, aiming for 2-3 sessions per week.
- Flexibility and Stretching

- Examples: Yoga, tai chi, or basic stretching exercises.
- Why It's Effective: These exercises improve range of motion, reduce muscle tightness, and promote relaxation. Flexibility exercises also help improve posture and reduce breathing difficulties.
- How to Start: Incorporate gentle stretches into your daily routine, especially after aerobic exercise or strength training.
- Breathing Exercises

- Examples: Pursed-lip breathing, diaphragmatic breathing.

- Why It's Effective: These exercises help improve your ability to control your breath, making it easier to breathe during physical activity. Pursed-lip breathing can slow your breathing rate and help you take in more air.
- How to Start: Practice these breathing techniques daily, especially before or during exercise, to help manage shortness of breath.

Tips for Exercising Safely with COPD

While exercise is incredibly beneficial, it's important to approach it carefully to avoid overexertion. Here are some key safety tips for exercising with COPD:

- Start Slowly and Gradually Increase Intensity

- If you're new to exercise, start with short, gentle sessions, and gradually increase both the time and intensity as your strength and stamina improve.
- Aim to exercise for at least 20-30 minutes, three to five times per week, but listen to your body and adjust accordingly.
- Warm Up and Cool Down

- Always start with a warm-up (5-10 minutes of slow walking or gentle stretching) and finish with a cool-down to prevent injury and allow your body to return to a resting state.
- Cooling down can also help ease any shortness of breath and promote recovery.
- Monitor Your Breathing

- Pay attention to your breath and take breaks as needed. If you experience significant breathlessness or chest pain, stop immediately and consult your healthcare provider.
- Practice breathing techniques like pursed-lip breathing to control your breathing during exercise.
- Stay Hydrated

- Drink plenty of water before, during, and after exercise. Proper hydration helps thin mucus and reduces the risk of dehydration.

- Wear Comfortable Clothing and Proper Footwear

- Choose loose, breathable clothes that allow for movement.
- Wear comfortable shoes with good arch support to reduce the risk of injury and improve balance.
- Use Supplemental Oxygen if Prescribed

- If you are prescribed supplemental oxygen during physical activity, be sure to use it as directed to maintain healthy oxygen levels during exercise.
- Talk to your healthcare provider about how much oxygen you should use while exercising.

Creating an Exercise Plan

Having a clear plan is essential for success. Here's how you can create a personalized exercise plan for COPD:

- Set Realistic Goals

- Start with small, achievable goals, such as walking for 10 minutes a day or performing a set number of repetitions in strength training.
- Track your progress and adjust your goals as you improve.
- Incorporate Variety

- Include a mix of aerobic, strength, and flexibility exercises to engage different muscle groups and keep things interesting.
- Choose activities that you enjoy and that feel manageable, whether it's a walk in the park, a dance class, or tai chi.
- Listen to Your Body

- Pay attention to how your body responds to exercise. If you feel overly fatigued, dizzy, or short of breath, take a break and reassess.
- Always consult your healthcare provider if you have any concerns about exercise or experience new symptoms.
- Consider Pulmonary Rehabilitation

- If you're struggling to start exercising on your own, consider enrolling in a pulmonary rehabilitation program. These programs provide supervised exercise routines tailored to your specific needs, along with education on managing COPD.

Staying Motivated
Staying motivated to exercise regularly can be challenging, but it's key to improving your health. Here are some strategies to keep you on track:
- Find an Exercise Buddy

- Exercising with a friend, family member, or support group can make it more enjoyable and help keep you accountable.
- Track Your Progress

- Keep a log of your activities, noting improvements in stamina, strength, and breathlessness. Celebrate milestones, no matter how small.
- Focus on the Benefits

- Remind yourself of the positive effects of exercise, like better breathing, reduced fatigue, and improved mental health.
- Make It Part of Your Routine

- Consistency is key to success. Set a regular time each day for exercise, whether in the morning, afternoon, or evening.

Conclusion

Exercise is one of the most effective tools in managing COPD. While it may take time to build stamina, the rewards are worth the effort. Regular physical activity can improve lung function, reduce breathlessness, and enhance your quality of life. Start slow, listen to your body, and gradually increase the intensity of your workouts. Over time, you'll feel stronger, more energetic, and better able to manage your condition.

Remember, the goal is progress, not perfection. Celebrate every step forward, and stay committed to incorporating exercise into your daily life.

CHAPTER 6: MENTAL AND EMOTIONAL WELL-BEING

Living with COPD affects more than just your physical health. It can also have a significant impact on your mental and emotional well-being. Feelings of anxiety, frustration, and even depression are common, especially as you adapt to the challenges of managing a chronic illness. This chapter explores the connection between COPD and mental health, highlights common emotional struggles, and provides strategies to help you maintain a positive outlook while navigating life with COPD.

The Emotional Impact of COPD

1. Coping with a Chronic Condition

Being diagnosed with COPD often comes with a range of emotions, including shock, denial, sadness, or anger. The realization that the condition is chronic and progressive can lead to feelings of loss or helplessness. These emotions are natural and part of the adjustment process.

2. Anxiety and Breathlessness

Shortness of breath is one of the most distressing symptoms of COPD. The fear of not being able to breathe can trigger episodes of anxiety or even panic attacks. This creates a vicious cycle, as anxiety can further worsen breathlessness, making it difficult to break free from the pattern.

3. Depression and Social Isolation

The limitations imposed by COPD—such as reduced physical activity, reliance on oxygen therapy, or difficulty participating in social events—can lead to feelings of isolation and loneliness. Over time, these factors may contribute to depression, characterized by persistent sadness, fatigue, or a loss of interest in previously enjoyed activities.

4. Guilt and Frustration

Some individuals with COPD, particularly those whose condition is linked to smoking, may struggle with feelings of guilt or regret. Additionally, frustration over physical limitations or reliance on others for help can further impact emotional well-being.

Recognizing Signs of Mental Health Challenges
It's essential to recognize the signs that your mental health may be affected by COPD. These include:
- Persistent sadness or hopelessness
- Loss of interest in activities you previously enjoyed
- Excessive worry or fear, especially about your health or the future
- Difficulty concentrating or making decisions
- Changes in sleep patterns (too much or too little sleep)
- Irritability or mood swings

If you experience these symptoms frequently, consider reaching out to a healthcare professional for support.

Strategies for Managing Emotional Well-being
1. Practice Mindfulness and Relaxation Techniques
Mindfulness and relaxation exercises can help you manage anxiety and reduce the stress associated with breathlessness.
- Breathing Exercises: Techniques such as pursed-lip breathing can calm your mind while improving your ability to manage shortness of breath.
- Meditation and Mindfulness: Apps like Headspace or Calm can guide you through mindfulness exercises, helping you focus on the present moment and reduce anxious thoughts.
- Progressive Muscle Relaxation (PMR): This involves tensing and then relaxing each muscle group to release physical and emotional tension.

2. Build a Support Network
Having a strong support system can make a significant difference in how you cope with COPD.

- Family and Friends: Share your feelings and experiences with loved ones. They can provide emotional support and help you feel less alone.
- Support Groups: Joining a COPD support group, either in person or online, allows you to connect with others who understand your challenges. The shared experience can be comforting and empowering.

3. Seek Professional Help

A mental health professional, such as a therapist or counselor, can help you work through feelings of anxiety or depression. Cognitive Behavioral Therapy (CBT) is particularly effective in addressing the negative thought patterns that can accompany chronic illness.

4. Stay Active Within Your Limits

Physical activity is beneficial for both physical and mental health. Even gentle exercises like walking, stretching, or chair yoga can release endorphins, improve your mood, and reduce feelings of depression. Consult your doctor about safe exercises for your condition.

5. Set Realistic Goals and Celebrate Small Wins

Setting small, achievable goals can help you regain a sense of control and accomplishment. For example, mastering a new breathing technique or completing a short walk can be significant milestones. Celebrate these victories to build confidence and motivation.

6. Educate Yourself About COPD

Understanding your condition can reduce fear and uncertainty. When you feel knowledgeable about COPD and its management, you're better equipped to make decisions about your care and face challenges with confidence.

Creating a Positive Mindset

Living with COPD requires resilience and adaptability. While it's natural to feel overwhelmed at times, there are steps you can take to maintain a positive outlook:

• Focus on What You Can Control: Concentrate on aspects of your life where you can make a difference, such as adhering to your treatment plan or maintaining healthy habits.

• Practice Gratitude: Take time each day to reflect on the positive aspects of your life. Keeping a gratitude journal can shift your focus from what's difficult to what's meaningful.

• Engage in Enjoyable Activities: Pursue hobbies or interests that bring you joy, whether it's reading, gardening, or spending time with loved ones.

When to Seek Help

If your emotional struggles feel overwhelming or persistent, it's important to seek help. Talk to your healthcare provider if you experience:

• Thoughts of self-harm or hopelessness
• Severe anxiety that disrupts your daily life
• A lack of interest in activities for more than two weeks

Your doctor may recommend counseling, medication, or a combination of both to support your mental health.

Conclusion

COPD may challenge your emotional well-being, but it doesn't have to define your outlook on life. By addressing mental health proactively, building a support system, and using effective coping strategies, you can maintain resilience and find joy in daily living. Remember, seeking help is a sign of strength, not weakness, and prioritizing your mental health is an essential part of thriving with COPD. You're not alone on this journey—support is always available.

CHAPTER 7: BREATHING TECHNIQUES FOR COPD

Breathing is something most people take for granted, but for those with COPD, breathing can become a challenge. Fortunately, there are several effective techniques that can help you manage breathlessness, improve your lung function, and enhance your overall quality of life. This chapter will explore various breathing techniques that can be incorporated into your daily routine to help you breathe more easily and reduce symptoms associated with COPD.

Why Breathing Techniques Are Important for COPD
COPD can cause the lungs to become inflamed and obstructed, making it difficult to breathe, especially during physical activity or flare-ups. Breathing exercises help:

- Improve Lung Efficiency

- Strengthen respiratory muscles, allowing for better lung expansion and air exchange.
- Improve the efficiency of oxygen uptake and carbon dioxide removal.
- Reduce Breathlessness

- Help manage the sensation of shortness of breath (dyspnea), which is common in COPD.
- By controlling your breathing, you can feel more in control during physical activity and stressful situations.
- Promote Relaxation

- Help reduce anxiety and panic, which can often make breathlessness worse.
- Encourage calmness, which is essential when managing a chronic illness.
- Increase Oxygen Supply

- By improving breathing patterns, these techniques help deliver more oxygen to your body, making daily tasks easier.

Effective Breathing Techniques for COPD

Here are some of the most beneficial breathing techniques that can help individuals with COPD manage their symptoms:

1. Pursed-Lip Breathing (PLB)

Pursed-lip breathing is one of the simplest and most effective techniques for controlling breathlessness and improving airflow. It helps keep the airways open longer, allowing you to exhale more air and remove trapped carbon dioxide.

How to Do Pursed-Lip Breathing:

- Sit up straight and relax your neck and shoulder muscles.
- Inhale slowly through your nose for 2 counts, keeping your mouth closed.
- Purse your lips as if you're going to whistle or blow out a candle.
- Exhale slowly through your pursed lips for 4 to 6 counts, making the exhalation longer than the inhalation.
- Focus on keeping your breathing slow and controlled. Repeat several times, especially during physical activity or when experiencing shortness of breath.

Benefits of Pursed-Lip Breathing:

- Helps you breathe out more fully, preventing air from getting trapped in the lungs.
- Reduces the effort required to breathe, easing shortness of breath.
- Can be particularly helpful during exercise or flare-ups.

2. Diaphragmatic Breathing (Abdominal Breathing)

Diaphragmatic breathing is designed to make use of the diaphragm, a large muscle located beneath your lungs, to improve airflow. This technique helps you breathe more deeply, increasing oxygen intake and reducing the effort required for breathing.

How to Do Diaphragmatic Breathing:

- Lie on your back or sit in a comfortable chair with your shoulders and neck relaxed.
- Place one hand on your chest and the other on your abdomen.
- Inhale slowly through your nose, aiming to expand your abdomen rather than your chest. You should feel your abdomen rise while your chest remains still.
- Exhale slowly through your mouth, pushing all the air out of your lungs. Feel your abdomen fall as you exhale.
- Continue for 5-10 minutes, focusing on deep, controlled breaths.

Benefits of Diaphragmatic Breathing:
- Engages the diaphragm fully, which is more efficient than shallow chest breathing.
- Reduces the work of breathing, making each breath more effective.
- Helps decrease stress and anxiety by promoting relaxation.

3. Box Breathing (Square Breathing)

Box breathing is a technique that helps regulate your breathing rhythm and reduces anxiety. It involves breathing in a controlled, deliberate pattern, often used in situations of stress or to enhance focus.

How to Do Box Breathing:
- Sit comfortably with your back straight and your hands on your lap or knees.
- Inhale deeply through your nose for a count of 4.
- Hold your breath for a count of 4.
- Exhale slowly through your mouth for a count of 4.
- Pause and hold your breath again for a count of 4.
- Repeat the cycle for several minutes.

Benefits of Box Breathing:
- Helps regulate breath patterns, making breathing more controlled.
- Increases oxygen levels and promotes mental clarity.
- Reduces anxiety and calms the nervous system,

particularly useful during flare-ups.

4. The Buteyko Method

The Buteyko Method is a breathing technique designed to retrain the body to breathe more slowly and gently. It is particularly effective for those with COPD and asthma by reducing over-breathing (hyperventilation) and improving oxygen levels.

How to Do The Buteyko Method:

- Sit or lie comfortably and relax your shoulders and neck.
- Breathe in and out gently through your nose, keeping your mouth closed.
- After a normal exhalation, hold your breath for a few seconds (start with 2 seconds and increase gradually).
- Breathe in gently through your nose once you feel the urge to inhale.
- Repeat this process several times, gradually increasing the time you hold your breath.

Benefits of the Buteyko Method:

- Helps reduce the tendency to over-breathe and lowers the risk of hyperventilation.
- Improves oxygenation by encouraging slower, controlled breathing.
- Can reduce symptoms of breathlessness and anxiety.

5. Breath Stacking

Breath stacking involves taking multiple small breaths, one after the other, to increase lung volume without straining. This technique can help people with COPD manage shortness of breath, especially during physical exertion.

How to Do Breath Stacking:

- Sit up straight and relax.
- Take a deep breath through your nose, filling your lungs.
- Without exhaling, take a second breath, filling your lungs more fully.
- Exhale slowly through your mouth, emptying your lungs.
- Repeat this process until you feel your lungs are adequately

filled, then rest and breathe normally.

Benefits of Breath Stacking:
- Helps to expand lung capacity and clear airways.
- Reduces the feeling of breathlessness.
- Can be used before exercise or during times of increased shortness of breath.

When to Use Breathing Techniques
- During Physical Activity

- Before or during exercise, use pursed-lip breathing to manage breathlessness. Diaphragmatic breathing can help you focus on breathing deeply and efficiently while moving.
- When Feeling Anxious or Panicked

- Use box breathing or diaphragmatic breathing to calm the nervous system during times of anxiety, helping reduce the perception of breathlessness.
- During Flare-ups

- If you experience a flare-up, use pursed-lip breathing to control your breathing and prevent panic. Diaphragmatic breathing can help you breathe more deeply and effectively.
- Before Sleep

- To help relax before bedtime, use deep breathing techniques such as diaphragmatic breathing or box breathing. These can help reduce the anxiety or stress that can exacerbate symptoms at night.

Creating a Breathing Routine
To reap the full benefits of these breathing techniques, it's important to practice them regularly. Consider the following tips for incorporating breathing exercises into your routine:
- Practice Daily

- Aim to spend at least 5-10 minutes each day practicing breathing techniques. This will help improve your lung function over time and reduce breathlessness when it occurs.

- Practice in Different Situations

- Try practicing your breathing techniques during different activities, such as walking, while sitting at your desk, or even during stressful moments to find which works best for you.
- Stay Consistent

- Consistency is key. Make breathing exercises a daily habit, and don't wait until you're feeling short of breath to practice.
- Track Your Progress

- Keep a journal to track your symptoms, including your use of breathing exercises and their effectiveness. This can help you determine which techniques work best for you.

Conclusion

Breathing techniques are essential tools for managing COPD and improving quality of life. By incorporating techniques like pursed-lip breathing, diaphragmatic breathing, and others into your daily routine, you can reduce breathlessness, improve oxygenation, and manage stress more effectively. Remember, consistency is key—practicing these techniques regularly will help you breathe easier and feel more in control of your condition.

CHAPTER 8: NUTRITION AND COPD: FUELING YOUR BODY FOR BETTER BREATHING

Proper nutrition plays a crucial role in managing COPD and maintaining overall health. COPD can affect your ability to eat, digest, and absorb nutrients, making it even more important to focus on a balanced diet that supports your respiratory and overall health. This chapter will explore the key aspects of nutrition for COPD, how to manage common eating difficulties, and tips for improving your nutrition to better manage your condition.

Why Nutrition Matters in COPD

When you have COPD, your body requires more energy to breathe, especially during periods of shortness of breath. As the disease progresses, you may also experience weight changes, difficulty swallowing, or a loss of appetite, which can make it harder to maintain good nutrition.

Good nutrition can help:

- Support Lung Function and Immune Health

- A well-balanced diet provides essential nutrients that support your immune system, helping to reduce the risk of infections (a major trigger for COPD flare-ups).
- Certain nutrients, like antioxidants, help protect the lungs from further damage and improve overall lung function.
- Maintain a Healthy Weight

- Maintaining a healthy weight is critical. Being underweight can lead to muscle weakness, which affects the muscles you use to breathe, while excess weight can place additional strain on the lungs.
- Reduce Inflammation

•   A healthy diet can help reduce the chronic inflammation associated with COPD, potentially decreasing the severity of symptoms and flare-ups.

•   Prevent or Manage Comorbidities

•   Many people with COPD also have other health conditions, such as heart disease or diabetes. Good nutrition helps to manage these conditions, improving your overall health and well-being.

Key Nutrients for People with COPD
Certain nutrients are especially important for people with COPD, as they can support lung health, reduce inflammation, and help with the management of symptoms.

1. Protein
Protein is essential for maintaining muscle mass and strength, including the muscles that help you breathe. Loss of muscle mass can lead to increased fatigue and difficulty breathing, as weak muscles require more energy to function.
Good Sources of Protein:
•   Lean meats (chicken, turkey, fish)
•   Eggs
•   Dairy products (milk, yogurt, cheese)
•   Legumes (beans, lentils)
•   Tofu and other plant-based protein sources
•   Nuts and seeds
Tip: Protein shakes or smoothies can be helpful if you struggle to eat solid foods or if your appetite is reduced.

2. Healthy Fats
Healthy fats, such as omega-3 fatty acids, can help reduce inflammation in the body and support heart and lung health. Omega-3s are particularly beneficial in managing COPD and may even reduce the frequency of flare-ups.
Good Sources of Healthy Fats:
•   Fatty fish (salmon, mackerel, sardines, tuna)
•   Nuts (walnuts, almonds)

- Seeds (flaxseeds, chia seeds)
- Olive oil and avocado
- Flaxseed oil and chia seeds

Tip: Include at least two servings of fatty fish per week to boost omega-3 intake.

3. Antioxidants

Antioxidants help protect the body's cells from damage caused by free radicals and oxidative stress, which are increased in people with COPD. These nutrients are essential for lung health and immune function.

Good Sources of Antioxidants:
- Vitamin C: Citrus fruits (oranges, grapefruits), strawberries, bell peppers, broccoli, Brussels sprouts
- Vitamin E: Nuts (almonds, sunflower seeds), green leafy vegetables, avocado, whole grains
- Beta-carotene: Carrots, sweet potatoes, spinach, kale, mangoes
- Selenium: Brazil nuts, tuna, sunflower seeds, eggs

Tip: Aim to incorporate a variety of colorful fruits and vegetables into your diet each day to ensure you're getting a wide range of antioxidants.

4. Fiber

Fiber is essential for digestive health, and a high-fiber diet can also help reduce the risk of constipation, which is a common side effect of COPD medications. Fiber also helps regulate blood sugar levels and supports heart health.

Good Sources of Fiber:
- Whole grains (brown rice, quinoa, oatmeal, whole wheat bread)
- Legumes (beans, lentils)
- Fruits (apples, pears, berries)
- Vegetables (broccoli, carrots, spinach)
- Nuts and seeds

Tip: Try to include a variety of fiber-rich foods in your meals and snacks to promote good digestive health.

5. Hydration

Staying hydrated is particularly important for people with COPD, as dehydration can make mucus thicker and more difficult to clear from the airways. Proper hydration helps thin mucus, making it easier to cough up and clear the lungs.

Tips for Staying Hydrated:

- Drink plenty of water throughout the day. Aim for at least 6-8 cups of water daily, unless otherwise advised by your healthcare provider.
- Limit caffeinated and alcoholic drinks, as they can lead to dehydration.
- If you have difficulty drinking water, try herbal teas or clear broths, which can also help with hydration.

Managing Common Eating Challenges with COPD

Living with COPD can bring several challenges when it comes to eating. Breathlessness, reduced appetite, or difficulty swallowing can make mealtime difficult. Here are some tips for overcoming common eating challenges:

1. Shortness of Breath While Eating

Eating can be a physically demanding activity for people with COPD, as it requires energy and coordination. If you become short of breath while eating, try the following strategies:

- Eat smaller, more frequent meals: This reduces the strain of eating large meals and helps prevent feeling too full, which can make breathing more difficult.
- Take breaks: If you feel out of breath while eating, take a short break to catch your breath before continuing.
- Sit up straight: Sit in an upright position to ensure your lungs can expand fully. Avoid reclining or lying down immediately after eating.

2. Loss of Appetite

Loss of appetite is a common issue for people with COPD,

especially during flare-ups. If you're struggling to maintain your weight due to a lack of appetite, consider these strategies:

• Eat nutrient-dense foods: Choose high-calorie, nutrient-rich foods to help you maintain weight, such as avocado, full-fat dairy products, nuts, and seeds.

• Consider meal supplements: Protein shakes or high-calorie nutritional supplements can be an easy way to get extra calories and nutrients.

• Focus on your favorite foods: Eating meals that you enjoy can help stimulate your appetite. Experiment with flavors and textures to make food more appealing.

3. Difficulty Swallowing (Dysphagia)

Some people with COPD experience difficulty swallowing, especially if they have other conditions, such as gastroesophageal reflux disease (GERD). To manage swallowing difficulties:

• Eat slowly and chew food thoroughly: Taking your time while eating can help prevent choking or coughing.

• Modify food textures: Soft, moist foods are easier to swallow. Consider pureed or blended foods if you have trouble swallowing solid foods.

• Avoid distractions while eating: Eating in a calm, quiet environment can help you focus on your breathing and swallowing.

Supplements: Do You Need Them?

While a balanced diet should provide most of the nutrients you need, some people with COPD may benefit from dietary supplements. It's important to talk to your healthcare provider before starting any supplement regimen, as some supplements can interact with medications or affect other aspects of health.

Common supplements that may be recommended for people with COPD include:

• Vitamin D: Many people with COPD have low levels of vitamin D, which is important for bone health and immune function.

- Omega-3 fatty acids: If you're not getting enough from your diet, omega-3 supplements may help reduce inflammation.
- Multivitamins: A daily multivitamin can help fill in any nutritional gaps.

Conclusion

Good nutrition is essential in managing COPD and improving your overall quality of life. By focusing on a well-balanced diet rich in protein, healthy fats, antioxidants, and fiber, and addressing common eating challenges, you can help manage your symptoms, reduce inflammation, and support your lung function. Always consult your healthcare provider or a dietitian before making significant changes to your diet or starting any new supplements.

Remember, nutrition isn't just about eating for survival—it's about fueling your body to feel your best and maintain your independence as you manage COPD.

CHAPTER 9: MANAGING COPD DAY-TO-DAY

Living with COPD means making adjustments to your daily life to help you manage your symptoms and maintain your quality of life. Each day can present new challenges, but with a thoughtful approach to daily activities, you can stay as active and independent as possible. This chapter will explore strategies for managing COPD on a day-to-day basis, from organizing your environment to managing your symptoms and finding support.

1. Creating a COPD-Friendly Environment

One of the first steps in managing COPD on a daily basis is making your home environment conducive to your needs. Simple adjustments to your living space can help reduce strain on your body and make it easier for you to breathe and move around.

Tips for a COPD-Friendly Home:

• Remove Clutter: Keep pathways clear to avoid tripping hazards and make movement easier. Organize your home so that items you use frequently are within easy reach.

• Maintain Good Air Quality: Dust, pet dander, and smoke can aggravate COPD symptoms. Use air purifiers, avoid smoking indoors, and make sure your home is well-ventilated.

• Create Comfortable Rest Areas: Set up a comfortable area where you can relax, read, or rest. Ensure it's easy to access, and consider adding a recliner or adjustable chair that allows you to rest without putting additional strain on your lungs.

• Use Assistive Devices: For tasks like cleaning or lifting, use assistive devices such as a reacher or a rolling cart to minimize physical exertion and reduce the risk of breathlessness.

2. Pacing Yourself Throughout the Day

COPD can make even routine activities exhausting, so it's essential to pace yourself and conserve energy. Rather than rushing through tasks, break them up into smaller segments and take breaks when needed. This allows you to stay active while preventing fatigue and breathlessness.

Pacing Tips:

•	Use the "Sit, Stand, Sit" Approach: For tasks like washing dishes, folding laundry, or cooking, alternate between sitting and standing. Sit down when you feel fatigued, then resume standing when you're ready.

•	Prioritize Tasks: Make a list of the most important tasks and tackle them first. Don't worry about completing everything on your list if you're feeling short of breath or tired—let less urgent tasks wait until later.

•	Plan Rest Periods: Build in short rest breaks throughout the day, especially after physical activities. Sit in a comfortable chair or lie down to rest and catch your breath.

•	Delegate: If possible, ask for help with tasks that cause you to feel winded, such as carrying heavy groceries or doing vigorous housework. Don't hesitate to reach out to a family member, friend, or caregiver for assistance.

3. Managing Symptoms of Breathlessness

Shortness of breath (dyspnea) is one of the most common symptoms of COPD, but there are strategies you can use to reduce its impact on your daily activities.

Strategies to Manage Shortness of Breath:

•	Practice Breathing Techniques: Use techniques like pursed-lip breathing or diaphragmatic breathing whenever you feel out of breath. These methods help you control your breathing, make each breath more efficient, and reduce anxiety.

•	Take Breaks During Physical Activity: If you feel short of breath while exercising or doing any physical activity, take a break. Use pursed-lip breathing to calm yourself, then resume when you feel ready.

•	Monitor Your Oxygen Levels: If your doctor has prescribed oxygen therapy, make sure you are using it as directed, especially during activities that might increase your shortness of breath.

•	Stay Calm: Anxiety can make breathlessness worse, so try to remain calm if you feel your breathing become labored. Focus on your breath and use relaxation techniques.

4. Staying Active and Exercising Safely

Although COPD may limit your ability to perform intense physical activities, staying active is essential for maintaining lung function, improving strength, and managing your weight. Regular exercise can help improve endurance, reduce breathlessness, and boost your overall health.

Exercise Guidelines for COPD:

•	Start Slow and Build Gradually: If you're not used to regular physical activity, start with gentle exercises and gradually increase the duration and intensity. Walking, light stretching, or low-impact aerobics are good options for those with COPD.

•	Incorporate Strength Training: Focus on exercises that strengthen the muscles you use for breathing, such as the diaphragm and chest muscles. Light weights or resistance bands can help build strength without putting too much strain on your body.

•	Try Pulmonary Rehabilitation: Pulmonary rehabilitation programs are designed to help people with COPD improve their physical fitness, learn breathing techniques, and manage symptoms. Ask your doctor if this program is right for you.

•	Monitor Your Symptoms: Pay attention to how your body responds during and after exercise. If you experience extreme shortness of breath, chest pain, or dizziness, stop exercising and consult your healthcare provider.

5. Managing Medications and Treatment Plans

Medication is an essential part of COPD management, and following your treatment plan as prescribed can help control symptoms, reduce flare-ups, and improve your overall quality of life. Be consistent with your medications and communicate with your healthcare provider about any changes in your symptoms or side effects.

Tips for Managing Your COPD Medications:

•	Create a Medication Schedule: Set a reminder or use a pill organizer to ensure you're taking your medications on time. If you take multiple medications, a daily planner can help you track them.

•	Inhalers and Nebulizers: Make sure you understand how to use your inhalers or nebulizers correctly. If you need help, ask your healthcare provider or pharmacist to demonstrate the proper technique.

•	Know Your Triggers: Keep track of what triggers your COPD symptoms (e.g., smoke, cold air, allergens) so that you can avoid them as much as possible. Be prepared with your rescue inhaler or medications in case of an exacerbation.

•	Discuss Side Effects: If you're experiencing side effects from your medications, talk to your doctor. They may be able to adjust your treatment to better suit your needs.

6. Getting the Support You Need

Managing COPD can be challenging, but you're not alone. Support from family, friends, healthcare professionals, and COPD support groups can help you navigate the ups and downs of living with a chronic condition.

Sources of Support:

•	Family and Friends: Having a support system is essential for maintaining mental and emotional health. Share your needs and challenges with loved ones so they can assist you in managing daily activities and provide emotional encouragement.

•   Healthcare Providers: Regular check-ups with your healthcare team are crucial for managing COPD. Your doctor, nurse, respiratory therapist, and dietitian can provide guidance on your treatment plan, exercise program, nutrition, and overall care.

•   Support Groups: Joining a COPD support group can help you connect with others who understand what you're going through. Sharing experiences, tips, and advice can provide emotional support and practical strategies for managing the disease.

•   Mental Health Support: COPD can lead to feelings of depression or anxiety, especially if you're dealing with persistent breathlessness. Seek mental health support if you're struggling emotionally. Cognitive behavioral therapy (CBT) or counseling can help you manage stress, anxiety, and depression related to your condition.

7. Monitoring Your COPD Symptoms

Regularly monitoring your symptoms is important for identifying potential flare-ups early and adjusting your treatment plan. Keeping a journal of your symptoms, medications, and triggers can help you and your healthcare provider stay on top of your condition.

Things to Monitor:

•   Breathing Difficulty: Note any changes in your breathing patterns, such as increased shortness of breath or wheezing.

•   Coughing and Mucus: Track any changes in the frequency or color of your cough or mucus. A persistent change can indicate an infection or flare-up.

•   Fatigue: Pay attention to how often you feel unusually tired or weak.

•   Medication Use: Keep track of when you need to use your rescue inhaler or nebulizer to assess whether your condition is worsening.

Conclusion

Managing COPD day-to-day involves making thoughtful adjustments to your lifestyle, creating a supportive environment, staying active, and keeping a close eye on your symptoms. With proper pacing, symptom management, and support, you can continue to live a fulfilling life while managing your COPD. By staying proactive and committed to your care plan, you can maintain independence and improve your overall well-being.

APPENDIX: ADDITIONAL RESOURCES AND INFORMATION FOR COPD MANAGEMENT

In this appendix, we've compiled additional resources and information that can help you in managing COPD, gaining further knowledge, and connecting with support systems. These resources include websites, organizations, tools for tracking symptoms, and more.

1. COPD Support and Advocacy Organizations

These organizations provide valuable information, support, and advocacy for individuals with COPD and their families. They offer educational materials, resources for managing the disease, and access to support groups.

- **American Lung Association (ALA)**

Website: https://www.lung.org/

The American Lung Association provides resources on COPD, including educational materials, advocacy for lung health, and access to local support groups.

- **COPD Foundation**

Website: https://www.copdfoundation.org/

The COPD Foundation offers educational resources, tools to help manage symptoms, and access to community support. They also provide COPD action plans and guidance on pulmonary rehabilitation.

- **National Heart, Lung, and Blood Institute (NHLBI)**

Website: https://www.nhlbi.nih.gov/

The NHLBI offers evidence-based information on COPD, including tips for managing the condition and the latest research on treatments.

- **British Lung Foundation (UK)**

Website: https://www.blf.org.uk/

The British Lung Foundation provides information on COPD, advice on living with the disease, and access to a variety of services for people in the UK.

- **Lung Foundation Australia**

Website:https://www.lungfoundation.com.au

Lung Foundation Australia provides comprehensive COPD information, support programs, and resources to help Australians manage their condition.

- **Canadian Lung Association**

Website: https://www.lung.ca/

The Canadian Lung Association provides evidence-based, user-friendly   patient resources

2. Pulmonary Rehabilitation Programs

Pulmonary rehabilitation is a medically supervised program designed to help people with chronic lung diseases like COPD improve their physical and emotional well-being. It typically includes exercise training, nutritional counseling, education on managing symptoms, and support from healthcare professionals.

- Pulmonary Rehabilitation Program Locator

If you're looking for a pulmonary rehabilitation program near you, visit the COPD Foundation's website https://www.copdfoundation.org/ or contact your healthcare provider for recommendations on local programs.

3. Symptom Tracking Tools

Keeping track of your COPD symptoms can help you and your healthcare provider monitor the progression of the disease and identify any changes that need attention. Here are some tools you can use to track your symptoms:

- COPD Symptom Diary

A COPD symptom diary is a simple way to track your symptoms, medication use, and triggers. You can use it to record information such as your breathing, coughing, mucus production, and energy levels. This information is helpful when discussing your condition with your doctor.

- MyCOPD App

There are several apps available for both Android and iOS devices that can help you track your symptoms, medications, and appointments. They can also provide educational content and breathing exercises.

- Peak Flow Meter

A peak flow meter is a simple device used to measure how fast you can exhale air. It can help monitor your lung function and track any changes in your airflow. Your doctor can recommend when and how to use a peak flow meter.

4. Breathing Exercises and Techniques

Breathing exercises are a key part of managing COPD. These exercises can help improve lung capacity, control shortness of breath, and reduce stress. Here are some of the most common techniques:

- Pursed-Lip Breathing

Pursed-lip breathing helps slow your breathing rate, making it easier to breathe out and keeping your airways open longer. To practice:

- Breathe in through your nose for 2 counts.
- Purse your lips as if you were going to whistle.
- Breathe out slowly through your pursed lips for 4 counts.
- Diaphragmatic Breathing (Abdominal Breathing)

This technique helps strengthen the diaphragm, the muscle that plays a key role in breathing. To practice:

- Sit or lie down in a comfortable position.
- Place one hand on your chest and the other on your abdomen.

- Breathe in slowly through your nose, letting your abdomen rise.
- Exhale slowly through pursed lips, allowing your abdomen to fall.
- The Buteyko Method

The Buteyko method focuses on slow, controlled breathing, which can help manage breathlessness and reduce hyperventilation. A trained therapist can guide you through the steps of this method.

5. COPD-Friendly Recipes

Eating the right foods can be a challenge, but a well-balanced, nutrient-dense diet is key for managing COPD. Here are a few recipe ideas to help you meet your nutritional needs:

- **Smoothies for Increased Calorie and Protein Intake**

Smoothies are a great way to pack in calories, protein, and nutrients if you have a reduced appetite or difficulty swallowing. Here's a simple recipe:

- 1 cup full-fat yogurt
- 1 banana
- 1 tbsp peanut butter or almond butter
- 1 tbsp chia seeds or ground flaxseeds
- 1/2 cup spinach or kale (optional)
- 1 cup milk or a milk alternative Blend all ingredients together for a high-calorie, nutrient-dense drink.

- **Salmon and Quinoa Bowl**

A rich source of omega-3 fatty acids, protein, and fiber, this recipe is great for lung health:

- 4 oz grilled salmon
- 1/2 cup cooked quinoa
- 1/2 avocado, sliced
- 1/2 cup steamed broccoli
- Drizzle with olive oil and lemon juice for added flavor.
- High-Protein Scramble

A nutrient-packed breakfast option:

- 2 eggs (or egg whites)
- 1/4 cup cooked spinach
- 1/4 cup diced tomatoes
- 1/4 cup shredded cheese
- Salt and pepper to taste

Scramble eggs with vegetables and top with cheese for a protein-rich meal to start your day.

6. Emergency Contact Information

It's important to be prepared for emergencies in case of a COPD exacerbation. Have the following information easily accessible:

- Primary Care Doctor's Contact Information
- Pulmonologist's Contact Information (if you see a specialist)
- Emergency Contact Numbers
- Emergency Plan for COPD Flare-Ups

Work with your healthcare provider to create a plan for managing flare-ups and exacerbations, including when to call for help, when to use your rescue inhaler, and when to visit the emergency room.

7. Further Reading and References

For those looking to dive deeper into COPD care and research, here are some books and articles that provide in-depth knowledge:

- Articles and Journals:

- The Journal of Chronic Obstructive Pulmonary Disease (JCOPD)
- COPD: Diagnosis and Management by Dr. Thomas R. Collins, available in many medical journals

8. Contact Your Healthcare Provider

Your healthcare provider is the most important resource in managing your COPD. Keep regular appointments, ask questions, and make sure you understand your treatment plan. If you're ever uncertain about symptoms, medications, or lifestyle adjustments, don't hesitate to reach out to your doctor, nurse, or respiratory therapist.

Conclusion

The journey with COPD can be daunting, but it's possible to lead a fulfilling life with the right knowledge, resources, and support. Use this appendix as a starting point for further exploration, and remember that the more informed and prepared you are, the better equipped you'll be to manage your condition. With consistent effort, a supportive team, and a proactive approach, you can continue to thrive while living with COPD.

Conclusion: Living Well with COPD

Living with COPD is undoubtedly challenging, but with the right knowledge, strategies, and support, it is possible to manage the disease and continue to live a fulfilling life. COPD may affect your breathing and daily activities, but it doesn't define you. By making small yet impactful changes to your lifestyle—such as focusing on nutrition, staying active, managing symptoms, and creating a supportive environment—you can take control of your health and improve your quality of life.

Throughout this e-book, we've explored the importance of understanding COPD, how to manage your condition effectively, and practical ways to handle the day-to-day challenges it brings. We've also discussed the importance of mental and emotional well-being, proper nutrition, and the role of healthcare professionals in helping you navigate your journey with COPD.

No matter where you are in your COPD journey, remember that you're not alone. With the right tools, knowledge, and support system, you can make informed decisions about your health and continue to pursue the things that matter most to you.

Key Takeaways:

• Education is Empowering: Understanding your condition is the first step toward better managing COPD. Knowledge about your symptoms, treatments, and coping strategies allows you to make informed choices about your care.

• Consistency in Care: Regular monitoring of your symptoms, adhering to your treatment plan, and maintaining open communication with your healthcare team are vital in preventing flare-ups and managing symptoms effectively.

• Support is Essential: Don't hesitate to reach out for help. Whether it's from healthcare providers, family members, or support groups, the emotional and practical support you receive will help you navigate the ups and downs of living with COPD.

• A Holistic Approach to Health: Managing COPD isn't just about addressing your lungs; it's about managing your whole body and mind. Nutrition, exercise, and mental health are all integral to improving your overall well-being.

• Adapt and Thrive: While COPD can bring new challenges, it also presents opportunities to make healthier choices, slow the progression of the disease, and live a more balanced life.

By taking proactive steps to manage your COPD, you can feel empowered to live well and thrive, no matter what stage of the disease you're in. Your journey with COPD is uniquely yours, but it doesn't have to be faced alone. You have the tools, resources, and support to live a full, vibrant life.

You've got this. With commitment, patience, and a positive outlook, you can keep moving forward, breathing easier, and enjoying life to the fullest.

Thank you for reading, and we wish you all the best on your journey to managing COPD and living well.